HERBAL REMEDIES

STRESS & TENSION

MERVYN A. MITTON

W. Foulsham & Company Limited
London · New York · Toronto · Cape Town · Sydney

W. Foulsham & Company Limited
Yeovil Road, Slough, Berkshire, SL1 4JH

ISBN 0-572-01254-3

Designed and Illustrated by Gecko Studio Services
Phototypeset in Great Britain by Input Typesetting Ltd,
London
and printed by St Edmundsbury Press,
Bury St Edmunds, Suffolk

Preface

During the early years of this century, by far the greatest majority of medicinal remedies available were based on herbal materials and, in fact, many of the formulae prescribed by doctors were the ones used with success in past centuries. Even as late as the 1940s it would probably be true to say that at least fifty per cent of a doctor's prescriptions would still have herbal materials contained in them.

During the sixties and seventies, the medical profession appeared to discard all of the older, proven methods of treatment in favour of new chemical-based drugs. The results of this revised thinking can be read about weekly in the newspapers, when they report side-effects – many of them very serious – from so many of these new and relatively untested medicines.

Within the last few years, however, there has been a dramatic resurgence of interest, both from the medical profession and the general public, in alternative forms of medicine – particularly herbs – and this book will help you to find your way through the many possibilities for safe home treatment. As a consulting herbalist at Cathay of Bournemouth, a firm established by my parents many years ago and now the largest retail herbalists in Great Britain, I can offer information and advice which is totally relevant and current.

Contents

Introduction

Conservative estimates put the number of prescriptions issued each year in the UK for tranquillisers at well over 20,000,000! This is a truly horrendous total, but to understand fully its implications you must also consider that knowledgeable medical opinion and statistics consider the following facts to be substantially accurate.

That 1 in 50 of the adult population is taking tranquillisers on any day of the year. That approximately 1 in 5 women and 1 in 10 men use tranquillisers in the course of a twelve-month period. That a 1982 report by RELEASE estimated that over 100,000 people – mostly women – are addicted to tranquillisers.

The dependence created by these drugs can often only be relieved by taking further quantities, and it is therefore not unusual to find people who have been taking them for many years. This is despite the fact that it is generally held that they all lose effectiveness after approximately four months of use – and some authorities say that this can be as short a time as two months!

The side-effects of these various tranquillising drugs can include anxiety, depression, sexual failure, apprehension, insomnia, and, for some, addiction. Additionally, it can often be dangerous to drive or work machinery after taking them, and if alcohol is taken at the same time it can enhance these various side-effects.

Withdrawal symptoms when a patient does decide to give up taking them can include sickness, nausea, headaches, violent shaking, loss of concentration and co-ordination, distorted vision and even suicidal tendencies.

Medical reports show that the commonest single reason for hospital admission is drug overdosage – as high as 15 per cent – and every year approximately 4,000 people die from taking too many drugs. The extent of the problem can be shown by the example of the City of Portsmouth who in April 1983 collected 3½ tons of unwanted drugs – including nearly a ton of tranquillisers!

The tragedy of all this accumulated misery and self-inflicted illness is that there are alternative forms of treatment which do not have the side-effects, and herbal treatment is at the forefront of these.

Tension and stress have always been problems, but never more so than with today's pace of life and breakdown of the family unit. With the long history of herbal medicine whereby the possible effects and benefits of a particular herb have been documented over many years, treatment can be tailored to suit an individual's particular needs and thereby help to reduce tensions and anxieties.

The important thing to remember is that, used correctly, herbs generally have no side-effects, they are not addictive, they do not cause depression and they do not require ever-increasing dosages to maintain their effect.

The recommendations in this book are all based on these known qualities of individual herbs and, in most cases, they can be easily prepared and taken at home. This home treatment approach is important, since experience has shown that many people who suffer disorders wish to try first to control the problem themselves.

This does not mean that where a serious medical condition exists, that it should be treated at home from the advice given in this book. In such a case, you should always contact your doctor immediately. However, where the pattern of the problem matches examples given, and where the advice is applicable, then herbal treatment could well be the answer.

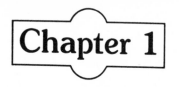

Chapter 1

Identifying your illness

Most people suffering from nervous tension will have sought medical advice and have had a correct diagnosis made of their particular problem. However, sometimes further complications arise, or the condition is not thought serious enough to worry the doctor, and it is for this reason that I show the various forms of this illness and their symptoms.

Many of the readers of this book will be dedicated already to the use of natural medicines, others will be seeking alternative treatments to conventional chemical medicines which they may have tried without success. The important thing to remember is that first you must be sure that you have correctly identified the problem – wrong diagnosis could possibly mean a worsening of the condition. Secondly, remember that herbal treatment is relatively slow acting and generally relies on a gradual build-up in the system. This makes it particularly suitable for problems such as nervous tension, since herbs are usually without side-effects, not addictive and compatible with each other.

ALOPECIA

This is another name for baldness and, obviously, there can be many contributory causes for the condition, including hereditary factors.

Nervous tension, or severe shock, can also have a serious

detrimental effect and often, when tension is present, the hair lacks lustre and becomes dry, brittle and comes out in greater quantities than usual.

Control of the nervous tension is of immediate importance together with suitable tonics to restore condition to the hair.

ANOREXIA NERVOSA

Usually this condition affects younger women and is 'triggered off' by a fixation concerning excessive weight. Symptoms show themselves as a very depressed appetite and insomnia.

Herbal nerve treatments can be of assistance, although in some cases psychological help is necessary.

ANXIETY STATES

Generally, this occurs when there is a state of mind where there is constant fear and worry concerning even the most trivial of everyday occurrences.

Herbal treatment can be very helpful.

DEPRESSION

Mental depression is a common illness and can show itself in different ways. Severe depression can make the sufferer feel that everyone is unfriendly and lead to immobilisation through fear. This is difficult to treat, and as serious problems, such as suicidal tendencies, are possible, psychological help is often necessary.

INSOMNIA

This is an interference with the normal pattern of sleep. Where tensions and anxieties are present they will often be main contributory causes and, therefore, a herbal nerve tonic will help to calm the nervous system and a herbal sleeping mixture will induce natural sleep.

MENOPAUSAL NEUROSIS

Severe shocks to the nervous system can cause amenorrhoea, or temporary cessation of menstruation. However, the menopausal conditions referred to here are mostly hot flushes and occasional irritability and depression which can occur.

A combination of St John's Wort and Squaw Weed (1 part of each made as an infusion) are old specifics for the condition.

NERVOUS DYSPEPSIA

Severe nervous tension can often lead to an increase in the amount of acid produced in the stomach, and interfere in other ways with the normal digestive processes. This can lead to indigestion, flatulence and similar discomfort. Effective herbal treatment will help to control these conditions and a herbal nerve tonic should be taken at the same time.

NERVOUS HEADACHE

This is one of the commonest types of headache and occurs when an individual becomes tense and worried. The strains of everyday life are common causes, although women undergoing menstruation are often sufferers.

Herbal treatment can be effective when these headaches are regular occurrences, and these are generally free of the side-effects of common chemical pain-killers.

NERVOUS TENSION

This is the most commonly encountered nervous problem and one which is likely to affect everyone, in various degrees of severity, at some time. Symptoms can include feelings of inadequacy, sweating and an upset stomach. If allowed to continue for a long period, poor hair condition, stomach ulcers and psoriasis can be brought about.

Herbal nerve treatment can be effective without further depressing the nervous system or being addictive.

MIGRAINE

It is generally accepted that there are two main causes which set off migraine attacks. The first of these is tension and worry, often allied with fatigue and eye-strain, while the second can often be linked with certain dairy foods, chocolate etc.

With the nervous type, our recommendations to patients usually include regular daily intake of a herbal nerve mixture and when an attack starts, this should be augmented for at least a seven-day period by a migraine specific. After a period of time I often find that both the frequency and duration of attacks can be greatly reduced.

TRAVEL SICKNESS

Nervous anticipation can often bring sickness to people undergoing a journey, or the tension, added to the motion of travel, can make the condition more severe. Ginger has always been known for its calming effect on the stomach and the formula for travel sickness given in Chapter 4 has had good results.

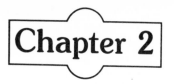

Chapter 2

Some commonly used drugs

This chapter outlines some main chemical drugs used in the treatment of stress and nervous tension, together with some of their side-effects. This information is given not to frighten people on these drugs, but to make them aware of all of their possible effects – however it should also be realised that not everyone taking a drug will necessarily suffer side-effects.

I believe that many doctors fail to explain fully to their patients the side-effects that can be expected from a particular drug or course of treatment, and this can cause great distress. This is usually a failure of communication since most drug companies advise doctors of the side-effects to be expected from their particular medicines.

Whilst there are other drugs used for stress and nervous tension which are not on the list and which are held to have less severe side-effects, it should be remembered that all chemical based drugs are expected to have side-effects.

Proprietary brand names are given in brackets beneath drug name.

AMITRIPTYLINE
(Saroten)
(Tryptizol)

May cause dryness of mouth and possible drowsiness. Dangerous during pregnancy.

AMPHETAMINE SULPHATE

May cause addiction.

ASPIRIN

May cause gastro-intestinal disturbance combined with blood loss. Care necessary for asthma sufferers.

CHLORDIAZEPOXIDE
(Librium)
(Tropium)

Some drowsiness and confusion may be caused. Possibility of dependency.

CHLOROTHIAZIDE
(Saluric)

May cause allergy and sometimes nausea.

CHLORPROMAZINE
(Largactil)

Care necessary in handling. May cause liver and blood problems.

CHLORPROTHIXENE
(Taractan)

Similar side-effects to Chlorpromazine.

DIAZEPAM
(Valium) (Atensine)

Possibility of dependency. May cause drowsiness.

GUANETHIDINE
(Ismelin)

Possibility of diarrhoea and general weakness.

GUANOCLOR
(Vatensol)

Care necessary for patients with liver problems.

GUANOXAN
(Envacar)

Possibility of liver damage.

HYDROXYZINE
(Atarax)

May cause drowsiness. Not recommended in pregnancy.

IMIPRAMINE
(Tofranil)

Slow acting and some side-effects possible.

IPRINDOLE
(Prondol)

Slow acting and some side-effects possible.

IPRONIAZID
(Marsalid)

Many dangerous side-effects.

LABETALOL
(Trandate)

Care necessary for asthma sufferers.

LORAZEPAM
(Ativan)

Possibility of some confusion.

METHAQUALONE
(Mandrax)

Some addictive properties.

METHYLDOPA
(Aldomet)

Possibility of drowsiness.

MIANSERIN
(Bolvidon) (Norval)

Possibility of reaction with other drugs.

NITRAZEPAM
(Mogadon)

Possibility of some addiction. Reacts with alcohol.

OXAZEPAM
(Serenid)

Possibility of some confusion and drowsiness.

OXYPERTINE
(Integrin)

Possibility, with large doses, of drowsiness, nausea and dizziness.

PERPHENAZINE
(Fentazin)

Care necessary in handling. May cause liver and blood problems.

PHENELZINE
(Nardil)

Many side-effects possible. May increase action of other drugs. (Even certain foods, particularly cheese, will react badly.)

PROCHLORPERAZINE
(Stemetil)

Care necessary in handling. May cause liver and blood problems.

RESERPINE
(Serpasil)

Possibility of depression, gastro-intestinal disturbance. Nasal congestion.

Chapter 3

Some problems which trouble sufferers

People who have had nervous complaints will not need to be told of the many side-effects which can occur as a result of the original nerve trouble. Even so, I often find that patients who come for consultations have not linked specific health problems with the original nervous condition. This means, of course, that when they are looking for treatment – either buying privately at a chemist or consulting their doctors – they are dealing with each illness as a separate issue, instead of looking for balanced overall treatment.

I have already mentioned vast numbers of prescriptions issued for tranquillising tablets, all of which can be addictive and have serious side-effects. These potential side-effects must be taken into account, since their effect is often to make the patient think they have a separate illness and, in turn, look for treatment for this. The result can be even more unnecessary drugs being introduced into the system.

Herbal treatment is generally without side-effects and after so many years of use, those that are present are fully understood. For this reason, herbal treatment is particularly suitable for nervous based problems, since it is not addictive, does not add to problems already present by causing depression, does not require continually increasing dosages to maintain benefits and is generally compatible with other herbal medicines and, indeed, with most chemical medicines which may have to be taken in addition.

There are three main ways in which nervous tension and anxieties can lead to additional illness; obviously, there can be others, but for someone considering home treatment, these are the three of greatest importance.

HAIR

That a severe shock can cause hair loss, or even a change of colour to white or grey virtually overnight, is well known, but unfortunately not many sufferers from severe nervous tension realise that it can also affect the general condition of their hair. I often find that there is a marked loss of condition when a person is under tension, usually the hair losing its gloss and becoming dry and brittle. Accelerated hair loss is often noticed when the hair is combed or brushed and baldness can quickly become apparent.

SKIN AILMENTS

Psoriasis can have a direct link with tension and, in fact, I very often find that its onset can be traced back to a severe emotional shock, such as a death in the family, or perhaps a divorce. Psoriasis is particularly difficult to treat since it often appears to clear, but at times of emotional disturbance perhaps even years later, may re-occur.

STOMACH ULCERS

When extremes of tension are experienced, particularly over a long period of time, the digestive processes of the stomach are disturbed. There are always amounts of acid present in the stomach which are necessary to help process food. But at times of tension, additional acid can be created which can attack the linings of the stomach and eventually cause ulcers to develop.

TREATMENTS

Specific treatments are recommended for the above health problems in both this book and in other volumes. However, the point I am making here is that to treat any of the above three without attention to the nervous problem which has originated them in the first place will not result in effective treatment. Herbal medicine has always had a complete approach of treatment for not only the effect but also the original cause, and it is for this reason that it is so often successful where other medicines fail.

Chapter 4

Herbal treatments and medication

The formulae in this chapter are all suitable to make at home following the given instructions and using quantities shown as percentages of the overall herb weight.

Ingredients should be available from herbalists and many health food shops – if any difficulty is experienced write direct to Cathay of Bournemouth Ltd, Cleveland Road, Bournemouth BH1 4QG or consult the list of suppliers at the back of the book.

INFORMATION ON THE PREPARATION OF HERBS

DECOCTIONS

The herbs are cut, ground up or bruised and covered with cold fresh water. This mixture is then boiled for up to half an hour, allowed to cool and then strained through a fine mesh. Allow 28 grams of the herbs to 568 ml of water (1 oz to 1 pint). This method is normally used when the herb is unsuitable to make as an infusion. The usual dose is approximately one small wineglassful three times daily.

INFUSIONS

Tea is made by the process of infusion. Prepare the herbs to be used and quickly pour boiling water on them. Allow the mixture to stand for about half an hour, stirring frequently and when ready strain off the liquid. Allow 28 grams to 568 ml of water (1 oz to 1 pint). The usual dose is approximately one small teacup or wineglassful three times daily; usually one after each main meal.

SOLID EXTRACTS

Start with a strong infusion of the herbs required and evaporate over low heat until a heavy consistency is obtained.

TINCTURES

This process is used for herbs and drugs which become useless when heated, or for those herbs which are not amenable to treatment by water. Tinctures are made with pure or diluted spirits of wine. Use 28 to 56 grams to 568 ml (1 to 2 oz to 1 pint). The dose varies according to strength of main ingredient.

SOME SIMPLE FORMULAE TO MAKE AT HOME

A GOOD GENERAL HERB MIXTURE FOR NERVOUS TENSION

Motherwort	1 part
Hops	1 part
Vervain	1 part
Lime Flowers	1 part
Scullcap	1 part

Make up as an infusion.

A HERB MIXTURE FOR NERVOUS HEADACHES

Betony	1 part
Scullcap	1 part
Valerian	1 part

Make up as an infusion.

A HERB MIXTURE FOR MIGRAINOUS HEADACHES

Rosemary	1 part
Valerian	1 part
Lavender Flowers	½ part
Lady's Slipper	1 part

Make up as an infusion.

A HERB MIXTURE FOR DEPRESSION

Oats (Avena)	1 part
Damiana (Turnera)	1 part
Kola	1 part
Rosemary	1 part

Make up as an infusion.

A HERB MIXTURE FOR NERVOUS EXCITABILITY AND ANXIETY

Cowslip Flowers (Primula)	1 part
Valerian	1 part
Lady's Slipper	1 part
Scullcap	1 part
Hops	1 part

Make up as an infusion.

A HERB MIXTURE FOR INSOMNIA

Hops	1 part
Pulsatilla	1 part
Cowslip Flowers (Primula)	1 part
Vervain	1 part

Make up as an infusion.

A HERB MIXTURE FOR MENOPAUSAL NEUROSIS

St John's Wort	1 part
Squaw Weed	1 part
Pulsatilla	1 part

Make up as an infusion.

A HERB MIXTURE FOR TRAVEL SICKNESS

German Chamomile	1 part
Ginger	1 part

Make up as an infusion

A HERB MIXTURE FOR NERVOUS DYSPEPSIA

Belgian Chamomile	1 part
Hops	1 part
Marshmallow	1 part
Lemon Balm	1 part
Meadowsweet	1 part

Make up as an infusion

A HERB MIXTURE FOR PSORIASIS

Mountain Grape	1 part
Burdock Root	1 part
Yellow Dock Root	1 part
Red Clover Flowers	1 part
Sarsaparilla	1 part

Make up as an infusion.

Chapter 5

Some recommended herbs

This section of the book will list in alphabetical order some of the herbs which can be used in the treatment of conditions mentioned earlier, together with other herbs of a generally beneficial nature.

A list of herbal suppliers will be given at the end of the section.

Mitton's Practical Modern Herbal, published by Foulsham, is recommended for a more complete list of medical herbs and their uses, together with much useful information.

ACACIA GUM (Acacia senegal)

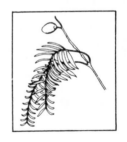

Also known as   Gum Arabic.
Found wild   North Africa.
Appearance   Round tears obtained from spring shrub. Cuts are made in the bark and the gum exudes and coagulates.
Part used   Coagulated gum.
Therapeutic uses   An excellent demulcent, often used to relieve catarrh and chest complaints.
Prepared as   Mucilage by combining with hot water.

ADDER'S TONGUE, AMERICAN (Erythronium americanum)

Also known as   Snake's Tongue.
Found wild   North America.

Appearance   Small bulbous plant with only two leaves; bright yellow lily-like flowers.
Part used   Leaves.
Therapeutic uses   Generally as a poultice for ulcers and skin troubles.
Prepared as   Poultice.

AGAR-AGAR (Gelidium amansii)
Also known as   Japanese Isinglass.
Found wild   Japan.
Appearance   Prepared from a compound of several different seaweeds into thin strips of about 30 cm long from dried jelly.
Part used   Translucent strips.
Therapeutic uses   Excellent for relief of stubborn constipation.
Prepared as   Powder.

AGRIMONY (Agrimonia eupatoria)
Also known as   Sticklewort.
Found wild   Throughout northern Europe.
Appearance   A strong-growing herb with green-grey leaves covered with soft hairs. Flowers are small and yellow on long slender spikes.
Part used   Herb.
Therapeutic uses   Dried leaves when infused make an astringent useful for diarrhoea; also as a tonic and diuretic.
Prepared as   Infusion.

ALDER, ENGLISH (Alnus glutinosa)
Found wild   England, Europe and North Africa.
Appearance   A small tree of distinctive appearance.

Parts used   Bark and leaves.
Therapeutic uses   The bark is used as a cathartic and the leaves to treat inflammation.
Prepared as   Decoction and poultice.

ALSTONIA BARK (Alstonia constricta)
Also known as   Fever Bark and Australian Quinine.
Found wild   Australia.
Appearance   Thick chocolate-coloured spongy bark from a moderate-sized tree.
Part used   Bark.
Therapeutic uses   To prevent recurring bouts of malaria and for quick and effective relief of most forms of rheumatism.
Prepared as   Powder or decoction.

AMARANTH (Amaranthus hypochondriacus)
Also known as   Love Lies Bleeding.
Found wild   UK and Europe.
Appearance   A common garden plant with crimson flowers similar to a coxscomb.
Part used   Herb.
Therapeutic uses   Treatment of diarrhoea and menorrhagia. As an astringent. Helpful in all cases of looseness of the bowel.
Prepared as   Decoction.

AMMONIACUM (Dorema ammoniacum)
Also known as   Gum Ammoniacum.
Found wild   Turkey and Iran.
Appearance   Small rounded lumps, pale yellow in colour, browning with age.
Part used   Gum resin.
Therapeutic uses   For respiratory troubles. Used in particular for the relief of catarrh, asthma and bronchitis.
Prepared as   Powder.

ANGELICA (Angelica archargelica)

Found wild   Europe and Asia.
Appearance   Plant growing from
one and a half to two metres high.
Parts used   Root, seeds and herb.
Therapeutic uses   For rheumatic
diseases, catarrh and asthma. A
stimulant and diaphoretic.
Prepared as   Infusion or decoction.

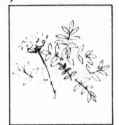

ANISEED (Pimpinella anisum)

Found wild   Europe, North Africa.
Appearance   An umbelliferous
plant with serrated leaves. Small
brownish-grey seeds.
Part used   Fruit.
Therapeutic use   A pectoral. Used
for cough medicines and elixirs.
Prepared as   Powder or decoction.

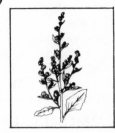

ARRACH (Chenopodium olidum)

Also known as   Goat's Arrach.
Found wild   Throughout Europe.
Appearance   A small inconspicuous
herb having an unpleasant odour.
Part used   Herb.
Therapeutic uses   As an
emmenagogue to bring on
menstruation. Also an effective
nervine.
Prepared as   Infusion.

AVENS (Geum urbunum)

Also known as   Colewort.
Found wild   Throughout Europe.
Appearance   Low-growing herb with yellow flowers.
Parts used   Herb and root.

Therapeutic uses   To stay bleeding and as a reliable tonic, particularly for women. Also used for treating leucorrhea.
Prepared as   Decoction.

BALM (Melissa officinalis)
Also known as   Lemon Balm and Sweet Balm.
Found wild   Throughout Europe.
Appearance   A plant up to one metre high, with a lemon odour.
Part used   Leaves.
Therapeutic uses   Most effective for the relief of flatulence and indigestion and induces copious perspiration. Can also be made up into a most pleasant and cooling tea.
Prepared as   Infusion.

BALM OF GILEAD (Populus candicans)
Also known as   Several other plants are known as Balm of Gilead.
Found wild   United States and Arabia.
Appearance   Strong gnarled shrub with feathery foliage.
Part used   Buds.
Therapeutic uses   Highly regarded tonic and diuretic. Excellent for chest troubles and rheumatic ailments.
Prepared as   Decoction or tincture.

BALMONY (Chelone glabra)
Also known as   Turtle Head and Snake Herb.
Found wild   North America.
Appearance   Low sturdy bush with oval dark leaves and white or pink flowers.
Part used   Leaves.
Therapeutic uses   Regarded as one of the best remedies for liver diseases. It is also antibilious, anthelmintic and a tonic.
Prepared as   Infusion.

BAYBERRY (Myrica carifera)
Also known as   Waxberry, Candleberry.
Found wild   Europe and North America.
Appearance   A medium-growing shrub with a profusion of large white berries.
Part used   Bark.
Therapeutic uses   A strong stimulant. A warming and effective deobstruent and cleanser. Also as a poultice for ulcers.
Prepared as   Infusion and poultice.

BEARSFOOT, AMERICAN (Polymnia uvedalia)
Also known as   Yellow Leaf Cup.
Found wild   North America.
Appearance   A tall branching plant found in loamy soil.
Part used   Root.
Therapeutic uses   For quick pain relief, as a gentle laxative for the aged and as a stimulant.
Prepared as   Decoction.

BETONY (Betonica officinalis)
Also known as   Wood Betony.
Found wild   UK and Europe.
Appearance   Plant growing to 60 cm. Long leaves with spiky flowers.
Part used   Herb.
Therapeutic uses   As a sedative, astringent and alterative. Of value for treatment for headaches and anxiety.
Prepared as   Infusion.

BIRCH, EUROPEAN (Betula alba)
Found wild   Europe.
Appearance   A strikingly handsome tree common on gravel soils. Distinctive black and white bark.
Parts used   Bark and leaves.
Therapeutic uses   Birch tar oil makes a soothing

ointment for skin disorders. The bark, as an infusion, is good for kidney stones.
Prepared as   Infusion and oil.

BISTORT (Polygonum bistorta)
Also known as   Adderwort.
Found wild   Europe and northern Britain.
Appearance   Low-growing herb chiefly found in ditches and damp places.
Part used   Root.
Therapeutic uses   Regarded as a cure for incontinence and as a gargle for sore throats.
Prepared as   Decoction.

BLACK ROOT (Leptandra virginica)
Also known as   Culver's Root.
Found wild   United States.
Appearance   A low-growing herb.
Part used   Rhizome.
Therapeutic uses   A blood purifying mixture. Also as a cathartic, diaphoretic and a liver stimulant.
Prepared as   Decoction.

BLADDERWRACK (Fucus vesiculosus)
Also known as   Seawrack and Kelpware.
Found wild   Around the coasts of Britain.
Appearance   A large trailing seaweed, dark green in colour.
Part used   Dried plant.
Therapeutic uses   To help reduce obesity also to tone up the system and clear the kidneys.
Prepared as   Decoction.

BLUE FLAG (Iris versicolor)
Also known as   Flag Lily and Water Flag.
Where found   Extensively planted in gardens throughout Britain.

Appearance   A beautiful plant with arching strap-like leaves and blue, white, yellow or multi-coloured flowers.

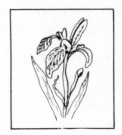

Part used   Rhizome.
Therapeutic uses   Principally as a blood purifier, also an alterative, diuretic and cathartic.
Prepared as   Decoction or powder.

BOLDO (Penmus bodus)

Also known as   Boldu.
Found wild   Chile.
Appearance   Medium-sized shrub with dark oval leaves and a strong lemon smell.
Part used   Leaves.
Therapeutic uses   As a liver stimulant. It also has antiseptic properties and is of value to sufferers of catarrh of the bladder.
Prepared as   Decoction.

BORAGE (Borago officinalis)

Also known as   Burrage.
Found wild   Throughout Europe.
Appearance   Bold, erect herb of strong growth. Small blue flowers.

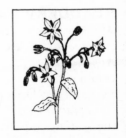

Part used   Leaves.
Therapeutic uses   As a tonic and stimulant. Also as a remedy for migraine and headaches.
Prepared as   Decoction or powder.

BOXWOOD, AMERICAN (Cornus florida)

Also known as   Dogwood and Cornel.
Found wild   United States.
Appearance   Small tree with rough bark and a profusion of pink spring flowers.

Parts used   Root and bark.
Therapeutic uses   As a tonic and stimulant. Also as a
remedy for migraine and headaches.
Prepared as   Decoction or powder.

BROOM (Cytisus scoparius)
Also known as   Irish Broom.
Found wild   Throughout Europe.
Appearance   A small graceful
arching shrub with profuse floral
display.
Part used   Top of each sprig.
Therapeutic uses   As a diuretic and
cathartic. Also used for the relief of
liver troubles and fluid retention.
Prepared as   Infusion.

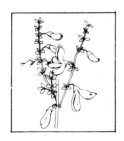

BUCHU (Barosma betulina)
Also known as   Bucco.
Found wild   Western coast of South Africa.
Appearance   Small procumbent herb growing in dry
places.
Part used   Leaves.
Therapeutic uses   Urinary and bladder troubles. Also a
diaphoretic and stimulant.
Prepared as   Infusion or decoction.

BUGLE (Ajuga reptans)
Also known as   Sicklewort.
Found wild   European woodlands.
Appearance   Diminutive herb with
distinctive square stems and blue
flower.
Part used   Herb.
Therapeutic uses   An astringent.
Prepared as   Infusion.

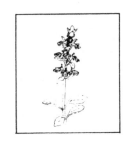

BUGLOSS (Echium vulgare)

Also known as   Viper's Bugloss.
Found wild   Europe.
Appearance   A sturdy herb with
blue flowers.
Part used   Herb.
Therapeutic uses   An expectorant
and demulcent. Excellent for gentle
bowel action. Also to clear phlegm
from bronchial tubes.
Prepared as   Infusion.

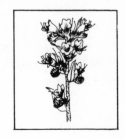

BURDOCK (Arctium lappa)

Also known as   Cockle Buttons.
Found wild   UK and Europe.
Appearance   Strong-growing plant
with large leaves.
Parts used   Root, seeds and leaves.
Therapeutic uses   Diuretic and
diaphoretic. For skin eruptions,
psoriasis, eczema and rheumatic
complaints.
Prepared as   Infusion or decoction.

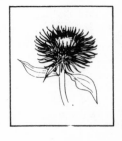

BUSH TEA (Cyclopia genistoides)

Also known as   Red Bush.
Found wild   South Africa.
Appearance   Small erect bush of striking appearance.
Part used   Herb.
Therapeutic uses   For kidney and liver disorders.
Prepared as   Infusion.

CANELLA (Canella alba)

Also known as   Wild Cinnamon.
Found wild   West Indies.
Appearance   Slender branching tree with light grey bark.
Part used   Bark.

Therapeutic uses   Stimulant tonic for the aged. Promotes digestion and elimination and prevents flatulence.
Prepared as   Decoction.

CARAWAY (Carum carvi)
Also known as   Caraway Seed.
Found wild   Europe and North Africa.
Appearance   A hollow-stemmed herb.
Part used   Fruit
Therapeutic use   As a flavouring.
Prepared as   Decoction or powder.

CAROBA (Jacaranda procera)
Also known as   Carob Tree.
Found wild   South Africa and South America.
Appearance   A handsome tree with lanceolate leaves.
Part used   Leaves.
Therapeutic uses   As a diaphoretic and diuretic. Also a safe sedative.
Prepared as   Infusion.

CASCARILLA (Croton eleuteria)
Also known as   Sweet Wood Bark.
Found wild   The Bahamas and West Indies.
Appearance   A diminutive tree.
Part used   Bark.
Therapeutic use   A tonic stimulant.
Prepared as   Decoction.

CATNIP (Nepeta cataria)
Also known as   Catmint.
Found wild   Britain.
Appearance   A procumbent grey plant.
Part used   Herb.
Therapeutic uses   Carminative and diaphoretic and has tonic properties. Also used for the relief of piles.
Prepared as   Infusion.

CAYENNE, HUNGARIAN (Capsicum tetragonum)

Also known as   Paprika.
Found wild   Hungary, also cultivated elsewhere.
Appearance   A strong-growing herb with large green fruits.
Part used   Fruit.
Therapeutic use   Rich source of vitamin C.
Prepared as   Powder.

CENTAURY (Centaurium erythraea)

Also known as   Feverwort.
Found wild   UK and Europe.
Appearance   Small pink-flowered herb.
Part used   Leaves.
Therapeutic uses   Stomachic, aromatic, bitter. For stomach upsets and anorexia nervosa.
Prepared as   Infusion.

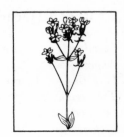

CHAMOMILE, BELGIAN (Anthemis nobilis)

Found wild   Belgium and France. Widely cultivated.
Appearance   Herb with double flowers.
Part used   Flowers.
Therapeutic uses   Widely used for women suffering from nervous upsets and as a tonic, stomachic and antispasmodic.
Prepared as   Infusion.

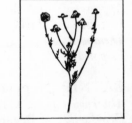

CHAMOMILE, GERMAN (Matricaria chamomilla)

Found wild   Europe.

Appearance   Herb with small cushion-like flowers in profusion.
Part used   Flowers.
Therapeutic uses   Excellent nerve sedative, carminative and tonic and as a poultice for leg ulcers.
Prepared as   Infusion and poultice.

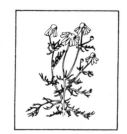

CHICKWEED (Stellaria media)

Also known as   Starweed.
Found wild   Britain.
Appearance   Small prolific weed.
Part used   Herb.
Therapeutic uses   A demulcent and to allay feverish conditions.
Prepared as   Decoction.

CHIRETTA (Swertia chirata)

Also known as   Indian Gentian.
Found wild   India.
Appearance   Small wiry herb growing in arid places.
Part used   Herb.
Therapeutic use   Tonic to restore flagging appetite.
Prepared as   Decoction.

CLOVER, RED (Trifolium pratense)

Also known as   Trefoil.
Found wild   Throughout Europe.
Appearance   A common clover.
Part used   Herb.
Therapeutic uses   Used as a sedative and to clear up nervous coughs, 'tickling' coughs and whooping cough. It is one of the best herbs to use for children.
Prepared as   Infusion.

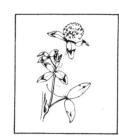

CLOVES (Eugenia caryophyllus)

Found wild   Zanzibar, Madagascar
and the East Indies.
Appearance   Beautiful evergreen
tree of majestic appearance.
Parts used   Flower, buds and oil.
Therapeutic uses   A stimulant and
carminative usually compounded
with other remedies.
Prepared as   Oil and spice.

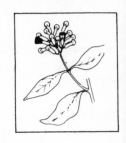

CLUBMOSS (Lycopodium clavatum)

Found wild   Northern hemisphere.
Appearance   Low spreading greyish-green plant usually
found near water.
Part used   Herb.
Therapeutic uses   Treatment of cystitis, kidney
complaints and urinary disorders. Also a sedative and for
stomach disorders.
Prepared as   Infusion.

COHOSH, BLUE (Caulophyllum thalictroides)

Also known as   Blueberry Root.
Found wild   United States and Canada.
Appearance   A gnarled, crowded shrub.
Part used   Rhizome.
Therapeutic uses   As a diuretic and emmenagogue also
as a vermifuge to expel worms. Aids rheumatic sufferers
and women's complaints.
Prepared as   Decoction.

COMFREY (Symphytum officinale)

Also known as   Knitbone and Slippery Root.
Found wild   Throughout UK and Europe.
Appearance   Fleshy-leaved plant about one metre high.
Parts used   Leaves and root.
Therapeutic uses   Helpful for treatment of internal

ulcers. For rheumatic pains and for arthritis and a poultice for treatment of bruises and sprains.
Prepared as   Decoction and poultice.

CONDURANGO (Marsdenia condurango)
Found wild   South America.
Appearance   Nondescript climbing vine found in heavily forested areas.
Part used   Bark.
Therapeutic uses   An alterative and stomachic. Helpful for treating duodenal ulcers.
Prepared as   Decoction or powder.

CORNSILK (Zea mays)
Found wild   South Africa and America.
Appearance   Maize.
Part used   Part of flower.
Therapeutic uses   Principally as a diuretic but also for pulmonary troubles.
Prepared as   Decoction.

COTTON ROOT (Gossypium herbaceum)
Found wild   Mediterranean islands and the United States.
Appearance   Twist of bark.
Part used   Bark of root.
Therapeutic use   Treatment of women's disorders.
Prepared as   Infusion and oil.

COWSLIP (Primula officinalis)
Also known as   Paigle.
Found wild   UK and Europe.
Appearance   Small wild flower.
Part used   Flowers.
Therapeutic uses   Sedative and hypnotic. Helpful in cases of insomnia and nervous restlessness.
Prepared as   Infusion.

CRAMP BARK (Viburnum opulus)

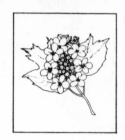

Also known as   Snow-ball Tree, Guelder Rose.
Found wild   Europe and America.
Appearance   Strong-growing bush with white ball-shaped flowers.
Part used   Bark.
Therapeutic uses   As a nervine for treatment of spasms and convulsions. Antispasmodic. Regarded as a safe children's medication.
Prepared as   Decoction.

CRANESBILL, AMERICAN (Geranium maculatum)

Also known as   Wild Geranium, Storksbill.
Found wild   United States.
Appearance   Shrubby small herb with blue flowers.
Parts used   Herb and root.
Therapeutic uses   Has quick styptic properties and is a tonic and astringent. Used as a treatment for piles and ulcers.
Prepared as   Decoction.

DAMIANA (Turnera diffusa)

Found wild   Southern USA and Mexico.
Appearance   Medium-sized shrub.
Parts used   Leaves and stem.
Therapeutic uses   Aphrodisiac. Tonic. Anti-depressant.
Prepared as   Infusion.

DANDELION (Taraxacus officinale)

Found wild   Most temperate climates.
Appearance   Common herb with long root, toothed leaves and bright yellow flowers.

Parts used   Leaves and root.
Therapeutic uses   As a tonic and diuretic and for liver and kidney ills. Roots frequently used for coffee as it contains no caffeine.
Prepared as   Infusion or decoction.

DODDER (Cuscuta epithymum)
Found wild   Throughout the world.
Appearance   A climbing parasite of the convolvulus family.
Part used   Herb.
Therapeutic uses   As a mild laxative and hepatic and for the treatment of bladder and liver troubles.
Prepared as   Infusion.

DOG ROSE (Rosa canina)
Also known as   Wild Briar.
Found wild   Europe and the Middle East.
Appearance   The wild rambling rose.
Part used   Fruit.
Therapeutic uses   The fruit yields ascorbic acid (vitamin C) of particular value when given to young children.
Prepared as   Syrup.

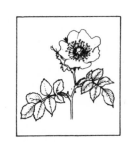

ECHINACEA (Echinacea angustifolia)
Also known as   Coneflower.
Found wild   United States.
Appearance   Herb of medium height.
Part used   Rhizome.
Therapeutic uses   Antiseptic and alterative and to help purify the blood. Also for typhoid.
Prepared as   Decoction.

ELDER (Sambucus nigra)

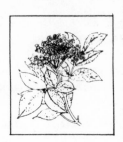

Also known as   Black Elder.
Found wild   Europe.
Appearance   A tall straggling shrub
with profuse crops of black berries.
Parts used   Flowers, berries and
bark.
Therapeutic uses   For colds and
influenza. As an alterative and
diuretic. It is a safe soporific and
induces healthy sleep.
Prepared as   Infusion.

EVENING PRIMROSE (Oenothera biennis)

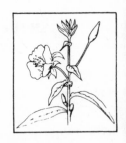

Also known as   Tree Primrose.
Found wild   European gardens.
Appearance   Small herb with a
delightful display of yellow flowers.
Parts used   Leaves and bark.
Therapeutic uses   As a sedative and
astringent. For the relief of female
menstrual disorders.
Prepared as   Decoction.

FENUGREEK (Trigonella foenum-graecum)

Found wild   Mediterranean area, North Africa and
India.
Appearance   Slender-stemmed plant.
Part used   Herb.
Therapeutic uses   As an emolient, a laxative and
expectorant. Can be applied externally to assist gout,
ulcers, wounds and boils.
Prepared as   Decoction and poultice.

FEVERFEW (Chrysanthemum parthenium)

Also known as   Featherfew.
Found wild   Throughout Europe.

Appearance   A small grey herb with hairy stems.
Part used   Herb.
Therapeutic uses   As an aperient, also used by women to bring on the menses. Now recognised as an aid to migraine.
Prepared as   Infusion.

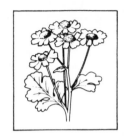

FIGWORT (Scrophularia nodosa)

Also known as   Throatwort.
Found wild   Throughout Europe.
Appearance   Herb.
Therapeutic uses   Aperient, also an emollient and demulcent and as a poultice for ulcers. Helpful for chronic skin complaints.
Prepared as   Infusion and poultice.

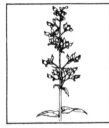

FRINGETREE (Chionanthus virginica)

Found wild   Southern United States.
Appearance   A small tree with inconspicuous white flowers. It has a very bitter taste.
Part used   The bark of the root.
Therapeutic use   Tonic, alterative and diuretic. Also for treatment of liver disorders, gallstones and jaundice.
Prepared as   Decoction.

GARLIC (Allium sativum)

Where found   Universally cultivated.
Appearance   Similar to a shallot.
Part used   Bulb.
Therapeutic uses   For treatment of dyspepsia and flatulence, also as a stimulant.
Prepared as   Juice and tincture.

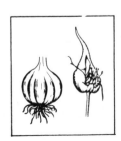

GELSEMIUM (Gelsemium sempervirens)
Also known as   Yellow Jasmine Root.
Found wild   Southern United States.
Appearance   Climbing plant with yellow flowers.
Part used   Root.
Therapeutic uses   Migraine, neuralgia, hypertension.
Prepared as   Decoction. (½ wineglassful 2 or 3 times daily.)

GENTIAN (Gentiana lutea)
Found wild   Alpine meadows.
Appearance   A plant with oblong pale green leaves and large, yellow, scented flowers.
Part used   Root.
Therapeutic use   Tonic.
Prepared as   Decoction or powder.

GERMANDER (Teucrium chamaedrys)
Also known as   Wall Germander.
Found wild   UK and Europe.
Appearance   Stemmed plant growing to about half a metre.
Part used   Herb.
Therapeutic uses   A helpful plant for the treatment of rheumatoid arthritis and gout. Has anti-inflammatory properties.
Prepared as   Decoction.

GINGER (Zingiber officinale)
Found wild   West Indies and China.
Appearance   About one metre high with glossy aromatic leaves.
Part used   Rhizome.
Therapeutic uses   Has stimulative and carminative properties and can be used as an expectorant and an aid to digestion.
Prepared as   Powder or decoction.

GINSENG (Panax quinquefolium)

Also known as   Panax.
Found wild   China and Mongolia.
Appearance   Erect-growing herb with fleshy leaves.
Part used   Root.
Therapeutic uses   Sedative, stomachic, aphrodisiac and tonic.
Prepared as   Decoction.

GOLDEN SEAL (Hydrastis canadensis)

Also known as   Yellow Root.
Where found   Cultivated in North America.
Appearance   Tall-growing herb with disagreeable odour.
Part used   Rhizome.
Therapeutic uses   For gastric disorders and as a soothing laxative and tonic.
Prepared as   Decoction or powder.

GUARANA (Paulinia cupana)

Also known as   Brazilian Cocoa.
Found wild   Brazil.
Appearance   A tall arching shrub.
Part used   Seeds.
Therapeutic uses   As a stimulant and for relief of headaches and migraine. Also used by women to bring on the menses and can be effective in the treatment of arthritis.
Prepared as   Decoction or powder.

HAWTHORN (Crataegus oxycantha)

Also known as   May Tree.
Found wild   Throughout Britain.
Appearance   A common small tree.
Part used   Fruit.
Therapeutic use   As an aid for heart conditions.
Prepared as   Decoction.

HOLLY (Ilex aquifolium)

Found wild   Throughout Europe.
Appearance   A small tree with
glossy leaves with a profusion of red
or yellow berries in winter.
Part used   Fruit.
Therapeutic uses   Mostly to relieve
chest troubles and laryngitis.
Prepared as   Decoction.

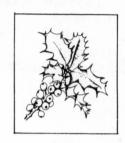

HOPS (Humulus lupulus)

Found wild   Europe and cultivated
in most parts of the world.
Appearance   A climbing vine.
Part used   Flowers.
Therapeutic uses   An anodyne for
the relief of pain. A tonic, an aid for
stomach disorders and to promote sleep.
Prepared as   Infusion.

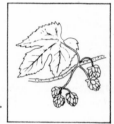

HORSERADISH (Cochlearia armoracia)

Found wild   Europe.
Appearance   A herb growing to one metre with a
pungent odour.
Part used   Root.
Therapeutic uses   Relieves flatulence and indigestion.
Promotes perspiration and is a diuretic.
Prepared as   Infusion.

HORSETAIL (Equisetum arvense)

Also known as   Scouring Rushes.
Found wild   Britain.
Appearance   A tall bold herb with cane-like appearance.
Part used   Herb.
Therapeutic uses   A powerful astringent and also a
diuretic. Excellent for kidney troubles.
Prepared as   Decoction.

HOUNDSTONGUE (Cynoglossum officinale)
Found wild   Britain.
Appearance   A medium-sized herb with long, strap-like leaves.
Part used   Herb.
Therapeutic uses   An anodyne for quick relief of pain. Also as a demulcent for soothing coughs and colds. Can also be used to reduce piles.
Prepared as   Infusion.

HOUSELEEK (Sempervivum tectorum)
Found wild   Throughout Britain.
Appearance   A small procumbent plant.
Part used   Leaves.
Therapeutic uses   As an astringent and poultice. Commonly used to soften corns and hard skin.
Prepared as   Infusion and poultice.

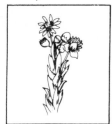

HYDROCOTYLE (Hydrocotyle asiatica)
Also known as   Indian Pennywort.
Found wild   Tropical India and Africa.
Appearance   A small plant similar to Angelica.
Part used   Leaves.
Therapeutic uses   As an aphrodisiac and also useful for treatment of urinary disorders.
Prepared as   Infusion.

HYSSOP (Hyssopus officinalis)
Found wild   UK.
Appearance   Small common field herb.
Part used   Leaves.
Therapeutic uses   Stimulant and carminative for bronchial and nasal catarrh. Also for anxiety states and tension.
Prepared as   Infusion.

ICELAND MOSS (Cetraria islandica)

Found wild Throughout northern hemisphere.
Appearance This is not a moss but a procumbent grey lichen.
Part used Plant.
Therapeutic uses For catarrh and bronchitis. It is a nutritive and helpful for digestive disorders.
Prepared as Decoction.

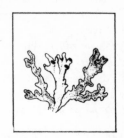

JABORANDI (Pilocarpus microphyllus)

Found wild Brazil.
Appearance A small herb.
Part used Leaves.
Therapeutic uses A diaphoretic and expectorant and is beneficial to asthma sufferers.
Prepared as Infusion.

JALAP (Ipomaega purga)

Found wild South America.
Appearance A robust climbing plant.
Part used Root.
Therapeutic use As a purgative.
Prepared as Decoction.

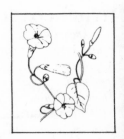

JAMBUL (Eugenia jambolana)

Also known as Java Plum.
Found wild East India.
Appearance A large spreading tree.
Part used Seeds.
Therapeutic uses Helpful to diabetics. Quickly reduces urinal sugar content.
Prepared as Decoction.

KAVA (Piper methysticum)

Also known as   Kava-Kava.
Found wild   South Pacific.
Appearance   Tall shrub.
Part used   Root.
Therapeutic uses   As a tonic and a diuretic. Helpful for the treatment of joint pains, rheumatism and gout.
Prepared as   Decoction.

KOLA (Cola vera)

Also known as   Kola Nut and Cola Nut.
Found wild   West Africa.
Appearance   A large tree of outstanding elegance.
Part used   Seeds.
Therapeutic uses   Celebrated for its aphrodisiac powers, it is also a nerve stimulant and heart tonic.
Prepared as   Powder.

LADY'S SLIPPER (Cypripedium rubescens)

Also known as   Nerveroot.
Found wild   Europe and USA.
Appearance   A delicate white orchid.
Part used   Rhizome.
Therapeutic uses   An effective nervine, valuable in cases of tension and anxiety. Tonic. Sedative.
Prepared as   Infusion.

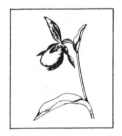

LAVENDER (Lavandula officinalis)

Found wild   UK and Europe.
Appearance   Familiar garden plant with grey needle-like leaves.
Part used   Flowers.
Therapeutic uses   Carminative and stimulant. Used for depressive headaches.
Prepared as   Infusion and oil.

LETTUCE, WILD (Lactuca virosa)

Found wild   Warm parts of Europe.
Appearance   A small plant of bushy
appearance.
Parts used   Leaves and juice.
Therapeutic uses   An anodyne and
sedative. Also useful to ease coughs
of nervous origin. Relieves rheumatic
pain.
Prepared as   Decoction.

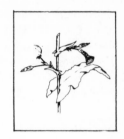

LIME FLOWERS (Tilia europoea)

Also known as   Linden Flowers.
Found wild   Throughout Europe.
Appearance   A graceful tree.
Part used   Flowers.
Therapeutic uses   A strong but safe
nervine for relief of headaches and
hysteria. Also as a stimulant and
tonic.
Prepared as   Infusion.

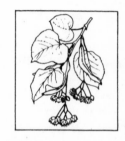

LIQUORICE (Glycyrrhiza glabra)

Found wild   Europe and the
Middle East.
Appearance   A strong-growing
perennial plant.
Part used   Root.
Therapeutic uses   In cough
medicines. As a demulcent and
pectoral and as a gentle laxative.
Prepared as   Decoction.

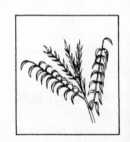

LOBELIA (Lobelia inflata)

Found wild   United States.
Appearance   A small trailing herb.
Part used   Herb.

Therapeutic uses   Stimulant, diaphoretic, expectorant.
Prepared as   Infusion.

LOGWOOD (Haematoxylon campechianum)
Found wild   South America.
Appearance   A massive tree.
Part used   Wood.
Therapeutic uses   To relieve diarrhoea and dysentery.
Also helpful for women's disorders.
Prepared as   Decoction.

MANNA (Fraxinus ornus)
Found wild   Mediterranean countries.
Appearance   Medium-sized shrub.
Part used   Sap from cuts in bark.
Therapeutic uses   As a gentle laxative for pregnant
women and as a nutritive invalid food.
Prepared as   Decoction.

MARSHMALLOW (Althaea officinalis)
Found wild   Throughout Europe.
Appearance   A strong-growing herb usually found in
watery places.
Parts used   Leaves and root.
Therapeutic uses   As an emollient and demulcent for
incorporation in cough medicines. Also for treatment of
cystitis and for soothing the alimentary canal.
Prepared as   Infusion and poultice.

MAYWEED (Anthemis cotula)
Also known as   Dog Fennel.
Found wild   Throughout Europe.
Appearance   A low-growing herb and common weed.
Part used   Herb.
Therapeutic uses   An antispasmodic with marked tonic
qualities. Excellent for migraine.
Prepared as   Infusion.

MEADOWSWEET (Filipendula ulmaria)

Also known as   Bridewort.
Found wild   UK and Europe.
Appearance   Long-stemmed herb
growing almost one metre.
Part used   Herb.
Therapeutic uses   Anti-rheumatic,
stomachic, astringent. Helpful for
severe cases of cystitis. Muscular,
rheumatic and joint pains.
Prepared as   Infusion.

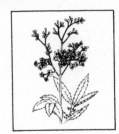

MOTHERWORT (Leonurus cardiaca)

Where found   A common garden
plant in Britain and northern
Europe.
Appearance   A pink-flowered
shrub.
Part used   Herb.
Therapeutic uses   A nervine and for
the relief of women's troubles. Also
a tonic and stimulant and helpful for
heart conditions.
Prepared as   Infusion.

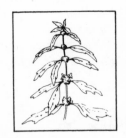

MULLEIN (Verbascum thapsus)

Found wild   Throughout Europe.
Appearance   Tall perennial cylindrical plant with a
tower of yellow flowers.
Parts used   Leaves and flowers.
Therapeutic uses   For lung and bronchial inflammations.
As an astringent, demulcent and pectoral.
Prepared as   Infusion.

NIGHT BLOOMING CEREUS (Cereus grandiflorus)

Found wild   Jamaica.

Appearance   A small branded cactus with large creamy flowers.
Part used   Plant.
Therapeutic uses   An effective heart stimulant and for relief of palpitations. Also a diuretic and helpful for prostate diseases.
Prepared as   Decoction.

NUTMEG (Myristica fragrans)
Found wild   Malaysia, Indonesia and the West Indies.
Appearance   Tall tree.
Parts used   Seeds and oil.
Therapeutic uses   Carminative, anti-emetic. Helpful in most cases of stomach upset. Can be used externally for the treatment of rheumatic pain. *Use in moderation.*
Prepared as   Powder and oil.

OATS (Avena sativa)
Found wild   In most temperate climates.
Appearance   A common farm crop similar to wheat.
Part used   Seeds.
Therapeutic uses   An effective nerve tonic and to allay spasms. Relieves rheumatic pain.
Prepared as   Decoction.

PAWPAW (Carica papaya)
Also known as   Melon Tree.
Found wild   Throughout sub-tropical areas.
Appearance   A tall tree (about seven metres) with boldly serrated leaves. Only the female produces fruit.
Part used   Papain from the juice.
Therapeutic uses   As a digestive aid, helpful for duodenal and peptic ulcers.
Prepared as   Powder.

PARAGUAY TEA (Ilex paraguensis)
Also known as   Mate Tea.

Found wild   South America.
Appearance   A dense shrub.
Part used   Leaves.
Therapeutic uses   Stimulant. Very helpful in the relief of
rheumatism and arthritis. Commonly used to make a
pleasant tea.
Prepared as   Infusion.

PARSLEY (Carum petroselinum)
Found wild   Europe.
Appearance   Bienniel umbelliferous plant with white
flowers and aromatic leaves.
Parts used   Seeds, root and leaves.
Therapeutic uses   As a diuretic and in the treatment of
kidney disorders, stones and gravel. Emmenagogue and
in the treatment of amenorrhoea.
Prepared as   Decoction.

PARSLEY PIERT (Alchemilla arvensis)
Also known as   Beakstone.
Found wild   Throughout Europe.
Appearance   A low-growing herb
with tiny green flowers. Not related
to common parsley.
Part used   Herb.
Therapeutic uses   For the relief of
bladder and kidney troubles and
helpful in dissolving kidney stones.
Prepared as   Infusion.

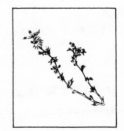

PARSLEY ROOT (Petroselinum crispum)
Found wild   UK and Europe.
Appearance   Small herb.
Part used   Root.
Therapeutic uses   Carminative, diuretic, emmenagogue.
Has useful anti-rheumatic properties.
Prepared as   Decoction.

PASSIONFLOWER (Passiflora incarnata)

Also known as   Maypop.
Found wild   Worldwide in warm climates.
Appearance   Climbing plant with purple fruits.
Parts used   Stem and leaves.
Therapeutic uses   Sedative, narcotic, antispasmodic. Useful for insomnia.
Prepared as   Infusion.

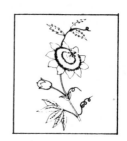

PENNYROYAL (Mentha pulegium)

Found wild   UK and Europe.
Appearance   Low-growing herb.
Part used   Herb and oil.
Therapeutic uses   Carminative, emmenagogue, stimulant, diaphoretic. This herb has always been regarded as reliable treatment for obstructed menstruation. Applied externally it is helpful for gout.
Prepared as   Infusion.

PEONY (Paeonia officinalis)

Found wild   Southern Asia.
Appearance   Beautiful perennial that bears vivid double flowers in profusion.
Part used   Root.
Therapeutic uses   Antispasmodic and tonic.
Prepared as   Infusion.

PEPPERMINT (Mentha piperita)

Also known as   Curled Mint.
Found wild   Europe and North America.
Appearance   A stately herb with purple-hued stems.
Part used   Herb.
Therapeutic uses   Stomachic and carminative. Relieves sickness, flatulence and indigestion.
Prepared as   Infusion.

PERIWINKLE, SOUTH AFRICAN (Vinca rosa)
Found wild   South Africa.
Appearance   Large trailing herb with profuse pink flowers.
Part used   Herb.
Therapeutic uses   Helpful for treatment of diabetes.
Prepared as   Infusion.

PICHI (Fabiana imbricata)
Found wild   South America.
Appearance   Herb of moderate growth with tiny leaves.
Parts used   Leaves and wood.
Therapeutic uses   Hepatic. Recommended for treatment of liver disorders. Also a stimulant and diuretic and helpful for catarrhal and kidney troubles.
Prepared as   Infusion.

PILEWORT (Ranunculus ficaria)
Also known as   Lesser Celandine.
Found wild   UK and Europe.
Appearance   A procumbent yellow-flowered herb.
Part used   Herb.
Therapeutic use   Excellent for treatment of piles.
Prepared as   Infusion and ointment.

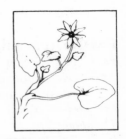

POPLAR, WHITE (Populus tremuloides)
Found wild   UK and Europe.
Appearance   Large tree.
Part used   Bark.
Therapeutic uses   Anti-rheumatic. Anti-inflammatory. Antiseptic. Beneficial to all cases of muscular and arthritic rheumatism.
Prepared as   Decoction.

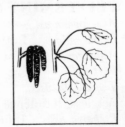

PRICKLY ASH (Zanthoxylum clavaherculis)
Found wild   North America.
Appearance   Medium-sized tree.
Parts used   Bark and berries.
Therapeutic uses   Diaphoretic, carminative, stimulant.
Helpful for circulation disorders associated with
rheumatism.
Prepared as   Decoction.

PULSATILLA (Anemone pulsatilla)
Also known as   Wind Flower.
Found wild   UK and Europe.
Appearance   A large weed with purple flowers.
Part used   Leaves.
Therapeutic uses   Sedative, nervine, antispasmodic.
Helpful for women with menstrual problems and also for
headaches associated with tension. Insomnia. Skin
eruptions.
Prepared as   Infusion (dried herb only).

QUASSIA (Picraena excelsa)
Found wild   West Indies.
Appearance   A tree of great stature.
Part used   Wood.
Therapeutic uses   As a tonic and also
effective for treatment of stomach
disorders. Helpful for cramp.
Prepared as   Infusion.

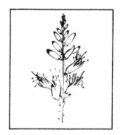

RED SAGE (Salvia officinalis)
Also known as   Sage.
Found wild   Europe and North America.
Appearance   A small herb.
Part used   Leaves.
Therapeutic uses   An astringent, helpful for sore throats,
quinsy and laryngitis.
Prepared as   Infusion.

ROSEMARY (Rosmarinus officinalis)

Found wild   UK and Europe.
Appearance   Evergreen shrub with
fragrant needle-type leaves.

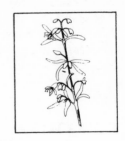

Part used   Leaves.
Therapeutic uses   Carminative,
nervine, tonic. Helpful in cases of
tension and migraine headaches.
Associated with hair care.
Prepared as   Infusion.

ST JOHN'S WORT (Hypericum perforatum)

Found wild   Britain.
Appearance   Sturdy yellow-flowered herb.
Part used   Herb.
Therapeutic uses   Diuretic. Expectorant, helpful for
coughs and bronchial ailments.
Prepared as   Decoction.

SAMPHIRE (Crithmum maritimum)

Also known as   Rock Samphire.
Found wild   England, particularly
in saline conditions.
Appearance   A small herb that
prefers shelter of rocks.

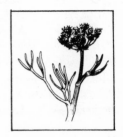

Part used   Herb.
Therapeutic uses   Diuretic with a
beneficial kidney action. Helpful for
weight loss.
Prepared as   Infusion.

SARSPARILLA (Smilax medica)

Found wild   South America.
Appearance   Bush.
Part used   Rhizome.
Therapeutic uses   Alterative, anti-rheumatic, antiseptic.
Helpful in cases of psoriasis and other skin ailments.

Long-standing treatment for severe rheumatism and
rheumatoid arthritis.
Prepared as   Decoction.

SASSAFRAS (Sassafras variifolium)
Found wild   Pacific coast of North
America.
Appearance   A shrub of average size
found in mountainous regions.
Parts used   Bark and root.
Therapeutic uses   Strong stimulant
and often used as an aphrodisiac.
Also effective for arthritis and
rheumatism.
Prepared as   Infusion.

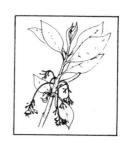

SAVORY, SUMMER (Satureia hortensis)
Where found   Commonly cultivated throughout the
world.
Appearance   A small shrubby plant.
Part used   Herb.
Therapeutic uses   For relief of flatulence and indigestion.
Also as a poultice to reduce inflammations.
Prepared as   Decoction.

SCULLCAP (Scutellaria laterifolia)
Found wild   United States.
Appearance   A herb of insignificant
appearance with pale blue flowers.
Part used   Herb.
Therapeutic uses   Famous as a
nervine and tonic, it relieves nervous
tension and St Vitus Dance. Scullcap
can be safely taken by persons of any
age under any conditions.
Prepared as   Infusion.

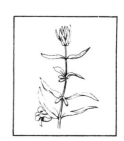

SENNA (Cassia angustifolia)

Found wild   Arabia.
Appearance   Tree of sparse growth
with distinctive grey-green leaves.
Parts used   Leaves and seed case.
Therapeutic uses   A safe laxative
without purging effect.
Prepared as   Infusion.

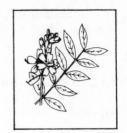

SHEPHERD'S PURSE (Capsella bursa-pastoris)

Found wild   Everywhere.
Appearance   Small insignificant
weed with little white flowers.
Part used   Herb.
Therapeutic uses   Diuretic, usually
for kidney and urinary troubles.
Antiscorbutic.
Prepared as   Infusion.

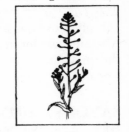

SLIPPERY ELM (Ulmus fulva)

Found wild   North America.
Appearance   A great tree of spreading growth.
Part used   Inner part of bark.
Therapeutic uses   As a nutritive for invalids. Also an
emollient and demulcent for healing burns and skin
troubles.
Prepared as   Infusion and powder.

SPEARMINT (Mentha viridis)

Found wild   Throughout the
northern hemisphere.
Appearance   Strong-growing
perennial herb.
Therapeutic uses   Stimulant.
Carminative. Suitable for the very
young and old.
Prepared as   Infusion.

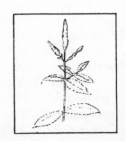

SQUAW WEED (Senecio aureus)
Also known as   Life Root Plant and Golden Senecio.
Found wild   UK, Europe and the United States.
Appearance   Common herb.
Parts used   Rhizome and leaves.
Therapeutic uses   Diuretic. Astringent. Tonic.
Menopausal neurosis.
Prepared as   Infusion.

SQUILL (Urfinea maritima)
Found wild   Southern Europe and North Africa.
Appearance   One of the lily family.
Part used   Corm.
Therapeutic uses   One of the most beneficial and much
used herbs. Expectorant. Helpful in relieving catarrh,
asthma and bronchial troubles. Also a cathartic and
diuretic.
Prepared as   Decoction.

SWAMP MILKWEED (Asclepias incarnata)
Found wild   United States.
Appearance   Medium-sized shrub of grotesque
appearance.
Parts used   Rhizome and root.
Therapeutic uses   It is a cathartic and an emetic.
Beneficial in the treatment of arthritis and stomach
disorders.
Prepared as   Infusion.

SWEET CHESTNUT (Castanea sativa)
Found wild   UK and Europe.
Appearance   Large tree.
Part used   Leaves.
Therapeutic uses   Astringent. Anti-rheumatic. Helpful in
cases of muscular rheumatism, lumbago and fibrositis.
Of specific benefit to catarrhal conditions.
Prepared as   Infusion.

VALERIAN (Valeriana officinalis)
Found wild   UK.
Appearance   A small herb.
Part used   Rhizome.
Therapeutic uses   Anodyne,
sedative, nervine. Excellent for
relieving nervous tension or nervous
debility. Promotes sleep.
Prepared as   Decoction.

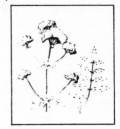

VERVAIN HERB (Verbena officinalis)
Found wild   UK.
Appearance   Small trailing herb.
Part used   Leaves.
Therapeutic uses   Tonic. Sudorific. Emetic. A very good
nervine to help depression and tension.
Prepared as   Infusion.

WATER DOCK (Rumex aquaticus)
Also known as   Bloodwort.
Found wild   Throughout Europe.
Appearance   One of the common
dock family.
Part used   Root.
Therapeutic uses   An alterative and
detergent. Helps clean and
strengthen gums and relieves mouth
ulcers.
Prepared as   Infusion.

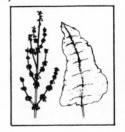

WILD CARROT (Caucus carota)
Found wild   UK and Europe.
Appearance   Small version of cultivated carrot.
Part used   Herb.
Therapeutic uses   Diuretic, carminative. Helpful in cases
of cystitis, bladder infection and gout.
Prepared as   Infusion.

WILD YAM ROOT (Dioscorea villosa)

Also known as   Rheumatism Root and Colic Root.
Found wild   North America and tropical areas.
Appearance   Tuberous plant.
Part used   Root.
Therapeutic uses   Anti-inflammatory, antispasmodic, diaphoretic. Helpful in the treatment of rheumatoid arthritis and muscular rheumatism. Leg cramps and intermittent claudication are two other conditions which can be beneficially treated.
Prepared as   Decoction.

WOOD SAGE (Teucrium scorodonia)

Also known as   Garlic Sage.
Found wild   UK.
Appearance   Small herb.
Part used   Herb.
Therapeutic uses   Respiratory infections, astringent, anti-rheumatic. This herb has been used for many years to treat respiratory infections and also rheumatic pain and stiffness.
Prepared as   Infusion.

YARROW (Achillea millefolium)

Also known as   Milfoil.
Found wild   Britain.
Appearance   A tiny herb.
Part used   Herb.
Therapeutic uses   A stimulant and diaphoretic. Excellent for treatment of influenza and heavy chest colds. Helpful for blood purifying.
Prepared as   Infusion.

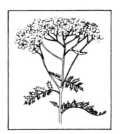

A guide to herbal suppliers

Herbalists tend to be rather thin on the ground and while your local health food shop should be able to assist with the more common dried herbs, specialist requirements often need specialist stockists.

The following list is by no means a complete one, but should be sufficient to cover most herbs mentioned in the book.

MAIL ORDER STOCKISTS

Cathay of Bournemouth Ltd
Cleveland Road
Bournemouth
BH1 4QG
(Free literature on request.)

Culpeper Ltd
Handstock Road
Linton
Cambs.
CB1 6NJ

MAJOR RETAIL OUTLETS

Bournemouth   Cathay of Bournemouth Ltd
Cleveland Road
Bournemouth
and
Hampshire House
Bourne Avenue
Central Bournemouth

Gerard House
736 Christchurch Road
Bournemouth
and
31 St Thomas Street
Lymington, Hants

Edinburgh   D. Napier & Sons Ltd
                   17–18 Bristo Place
                   Edinburgh

Jersey   Norwegian Health Salon
                   6a La Motte Street
                   Jersey
                   Channel Islands

London   G. Baldwin
                   171–173 Walworth Road
                   London
                   SE17

                   Neal's Yard Apothecary
                   Neal's Yard
                   Covent Garden
                   London
                   WC2

Ryde   The Grail Pharmacy
                   The Collonade
                   Lind Street
                   Ryde
                   Isle of Wight

Sheffield   Wickers Health Stores
                   195 Cattle Market
                   Sheffield

Southampton   Cathay of Bournemouth Ltd
                   32–33 Hanover Buildings
                   Central Southampton

Culpeper Herbal Shops can be found in nine major towns,
including three in London.

Glossary of common medical terms

Very often when reading, or on having a medical consultation, words are used which may not be familiar. This short list will help to make some of the more common ones a little clearer.

Alterative   Any substance that can beneficially alter the condition of a patient.

Amenorrhoea   Cessation of the menstrual flow.

Anodyne   Any substance which eases pain.

Antiseptic   Any substance that prevents putrefaction.

Antispasmodic   Any substance that prevents or relieves spasms.

Anthelmintic   Any herb acting against intestinal worms.

Aperient   Any substance producing the natural evacuation of the bowels.

Aphrodisiac   Any substance that stimulates sexual functions.

Astringent   Any substance which causes contraction of body tissues.

Cardiac   Any condition affecting or pertaining to the heart.

Carminative   Any substance that relieves pain caused by flatulence.

Cathartic   Any substance that induces stimulation of bowel action; rather stronger than aperients.

Corrective   Any substance that restores normal conditions.